Michele Maia Pontes

Effects of a dance program on senescence

Michele Maia Pontes

Effects of a dance program on senescence

With movements similar to the activities of daily living of the elderly

ScienciaScripts

Imprint

Any brand names and product names mentioned in this book are subject to trademark, brand or patent protection and are trademarks or registered trademarks of their respective holders. The use of brand names, product names, common names, trade names, product descriptions etc. even without a particular marking in this work is in no way to be construed to mean that such names may be regarded as unrestricted in respect of trademark and brand protection legislation and could thus be used by anyone.

Cover image: www.ingimage.com

This book is a translation from the original published under ISBN 978-613-9-67199-1.

Publisher:
Sciencia Scripts
is a trademark of
Dodo Books Indian Ocean Ltd. and OmniScriptum S.R.L publishing group

120 High Road, East Finchley, London, N2 9ED, United Kingdom
Str. Armeneasca 28/1, office 1, Chisinau MD-2012, Republic of Moldova, Europe
Printed at: see last page
ISBN: 978-620-8-15567-4

SUMMARY

SUMMARY

Population ageing is a worldwide phenomenon, and this growth requires attention because senescence causes a decline in physical functions, which can lead to dependency. Physical activity appears to be an instrument for minimizing or even remedying functional incapacities, such as dance. The aim of this study was to analyze the effects of a dance program with movements similar to activities of daily living on the functional response of the elderly. Fifty-nine elderly people took part in the study, with an average age of 68±4 years. The results showed significant positive changes in lower limb strength (25% increase) and upper limb strength (24%), aerobic endurance (21%) and balance (15%). With regard to flexibility, there was no statistically significant difference (p≤0.05), but we observed its maintenance. We conclude that the functional dance program promoted the maintenance and significant gains in the motor functions of the elderly.

Keyword: Ageing. Physical Activities. Dance

1. INTRODUCTION

Population ageing is currently a worldwide phenomenon, especially in developing countries such as Brazil, where the demographic transition is occurring at an accelerated rate (DUCA HALLAL; SILVA; 2009). Alves (2008) states that the demographic transition begins with a reduction in mortality rates and, after a while, with a fall in birth rates, causing significant changes in the age structure of the population. Data from the IBGE (2008) show that Brazil should have the sixth oldest population on the planet by 2025, with 34 million people over the age of 70, which will represent 14% of the Brazilian population. Miranda et al. (2016) reflect that the country is ageing at a rapid pace. The changes in the population structure are clear and irreversible. This data deserves special attention, as it makes us reflect on aggravating factors: fewer people working and more retired elderly people, which has a significant impact on the economy and consequently on the family structure, in addition to the fact that ageing causes loss of functional capacities, which can lead to dependency.

According to Pereira (2012), the human ageing process is characterized by a series of changes in biological, psychological and social functions, which occur progressively, leading to losses and/or reductions in the ability to perform certain tasks.

Correa, Oliveira and Bassani (2018) argue that the various meanings attributed to ageing challenge the understanding of the ways in which an elderly person represents themselves in the world, which can lead to the idea that Minayo and Coimbra (2002) called "social weight", significantly affecting the elderly person's way of living. Because faced with these social representations of ageing, the elderly person starts to feel demeaned. Silva; Scorsolini and Santos (2013) add to this discourse by saying that these representations become an obstacle even in family life, in their relationships, generating conflicts, which can lead to the elderly being placed in a Long-Stay Institution for the Elderly by the will of the elderly person or by determination of family members. Correa; Oliveira and Bassani (2018, p.167) describe these institutions as "(...) spaces that offer assistance to the elderly, seeking to guarantee their physical, psychological and social well-being in line with the Statute of the Elderly and other policies aimed at the elderly". But how do you preserve all these aspects away from your real home, away from the people with whom your history was built? The elderly face new challenges Freitas, Queiroz and Sousa (2010) point out that, in situations of institutionalization, illnesses become frequent and limiting obstacles. This is perhaps more accentuated by the fact that people miss their homes, and long-stay institutions follow common patterns of living together, which deviate from people's unique routine habits, and this can generate unease in anyone.

In order to better deal with this paradigm, parents, according to Miranda et al (2016), have been trying to better understand this phenomenon called ageing and, according to Kalache (2008), "keep their elderly citizens socially and economically integrated and independent".

The United Nations Population Fund, in its report on ageing in the 21st century, pointed out that although many countries have made important progress in adapting their policies and laws, more efforts need to be directed towards ensuring that older people can reach their potential.

We can see that the public health and social security systems deserve special attention at this time.

Although Miranda et al (2016, p.508) reminds us:

Getting older doesn't necessarily mean getting sick. Unless there is an associated disease, ageing is associated with a good level of health. In addition, advances in the field of health and technology have enabled people with access to adequate public or private services to enjoy a better quality of life during this phase.

Lima-Costa et al (2011) in their study on the health trends of the elderly Brazilian population, using data from the National Household Sample Survey, identified improvements in some aspects of the health of the elderly, such as a reduction in hospitalizations. For the authors, the results corroborate the expansion of primary care in the country.

Miranda et al (2016) show in another study that in 2013, hospital care for the elderly population grew in relation to public spending on hospitalizations, but this increase compared to the percentage of the elderly population is a small growth.

Above all, Matsudo (2010) reveals some biological changes that occur in the body during senescence, such as a reduction in the strength of the upper and lower limbs, sensory losses that affect balance, a reduction in hip, spinal and ankle flexion, a decline in maximum oxygen consumption and a loss of lean mass.

With reduced physical capacities we have limitations in body movement, affecting the motor repertoire and impairing simple daily activities.

According to Couto and Ovando (2010) among the elderly, chronic conditions tend to manifest themselves in a more significant way, due to the functional declines of aging, thus, these conditions tend to significantly compromise quality of life, affecting performance in activities of daily living, which are subdivided into Basic Activities of Daily Living (BADL), Instrumental Activities of Daily Living (IADL) and Advanced Activities of Daily Living (AADL). The American Geriatrics Society (2009) classifies activities of daily living in the same way and explains each one: ABDV; are the activities of self-care, AIVD; encompass ABDV and include tasks essential for maintaining independence, AAVD; refer to the functions necessary to live alone, being specific to each individual, they include the maintenance of occupational functions, recreation and the provision of community services.

Functional disabilities resulting from the ageing process progress significantly, so attention is essential as soon as the first difficulties arise.

According to Duca, Hallal and Silva (2009) functional incapacity is characterized as any restriction to perform an activity considered normal within the human extension. Depending on the degree of impairment in functional capacities, the elderly person may be partially or totally dependent on others to carry out daily activities.

According to Borges and Moreira (2009) disability makes the elderly dependent on other people for simple tasks such as leaving the house alone. The tendency is for this condition to worsen, progressing to self-care activities such as bathing or going to the toilet alone. When elderly people become dependent on others for their tasks, especially self-care, they lose their functional autonomy and feel devalued, which impacts on their quality of life.

Physical activity appears to be an excellent tool for improving the quality of life of the elderly, because through it we can minimize or even remedy the difficulties in performing everyday tasks and offer the individual functional autonomy (BORGES, MOREIRA, 2009).

Matsudo (2010) reveals the effects of practicing physical activity in the elderly: controlling or reducing body fat, maintaining or increasing muscle mass, muscle strength, strengthening connective tissue, improving flexibility, increasing circulating blood volume, reducing heart rate and blood pressure at rest, improved HDL levels, lower levels of triglycerides, total cholesterol and LDL, lower glucose levels, reduced risk of cardiovascular disease, thromboembolic stroke, hypertension, type II diabetes, osteoporosis and obesity. In addition to cognitive and psychosocial benefits such as improved self-concept, self-esteem, body image, mood, muscle tension and insomnia, among others.

According to Borges and Moreira (2009) many elderly people are already seeking a healthier, more active and independent life. Currently, there is an increase in programs related to promoting the health and well-being of these individuals. Among these programs is the practice of physical activities through sports, dance, strength training or recreational activities, all of which bring benefits in some way.

Among the various forms of physical exercise, dance is a valuable tool for the elderly. According to Golin (2005), dance offers us many advantages in society, as it allows us to express our feelings, body awareness, self-knowledge, knowledge of others, socialization, and it helps us both physically and psychologically. For Carla et al (2013), dance contributes significantly to the improvement and/or maintenance of various dimensions that are included in the term "quality of life", including social integration, adaptation to pre-existing conditions and functional ability.

Tavares (2001) believes that dance is linked to the need to express feelings, desires, realities and dreams, and that all these emotions are expressed in the body's postural model, thus judging dance movement not just as the displacement of a body in space, but as a process capable of taking man to infinite possibilities of transformation.

Systematic studies on body image and dance are recent and most of them emphasize its role in the biopsychosocial process (TAVARES, 2001). According to Marciano and Barbosa (2009), body image is the way in which our body appears to ourselves. It is the mental representation of our own body. The perception of body image can be defined as an illustration in the mind of the size, image and shape of the body, as well as the feelings related to these characteristics and the parts that make it up.

Tavares (2003) says that early childhood experiences are fundamental in the process of developing body image, but we never stop having experiences and exploring our bodies. This conception points to the significance of our bodily experiences throughout our lives, and also highlights the importance of bodily interventions in the process of people's development, from birth to old age.

Understanding the aging process and creating interventions that offer a better quality of life for the elderly population is fundamental. Strategies to keep them independent for as long as possible become an important prevention tool for society and health professionals from a collective health perspective. At this stage of life, the functional decline of the body can compromise the social life of the elderly and damage their self-esteem.

In this way, dance plays an important role in the elderly population, enabling interaction between the individuals who practice it, awakening the pleasure of exploring feelings, letting them expand with gestures and movements.

In view of the above, the objective of this study will be to verify the degree of dependence of the elderly who practice a physical activity program at the IPGG (Instituto Paulista de Geriatria e Gerontologia) located in Sao Miguel Paulista, and to analyze the effects of a dance program with diversified rhythms and movements similar to activities of daily living on the functional response and body perception of the elderly.

2. SPECIFIC OBJECTIVES

V To verify the degree of dependence of the elderly who practice a physical activity program at the IPGG (Instituto Paulista de Geriatria e Gerontologia) in basic activities of daily living (ABVD), instrumental activities of daily living (AIDV) and advanced activities of daily living (AAVD);

S Teaching dance classes to people over 60 for a period of 12 consecutive weeks;

V Evaluate the effects of dance classes on the variables:

> Balance;

> Muscle strength;

> Flexibility;

> Aerobic endurance;

3.   EXPECTED RESULTS

Analyzing the above context, we expect to find a significant number of elderly people who are independent in their daily activities, because they are physically active and attend the physical activity program. We intend to verify a significant improvement in motor skills: balance; flexibility; aerobic endurance; upper and lower limb strength, after the 12-week dance program, as well as measuring the level of body satisfaction of the elderly before and after the intervention.

4. METHOD

This research is of a descriptive experimental nature because its premise is to seek to solve problems by improving practices through observation, analysis and objective descriptions, and content validation (THOMAS; NELSON; SILVERMAN, 2007). The purpose of descriptive research is to observe, record and analyze phenomena without, however, going into the content. It is a descriptive experimental type with a quantitative approach because it observes facts and phenomena, collects data on them and, finally, analyzes and interprets this data, based on a consistent theoretical foundation, with the aim of understanding and explaining the hypothesis raised.

4.1 Subjects

Fifty-nine elderly people aged 60 or over, belonging to a gymnastics group at the IPGG, called Maintenance Gymnastics, took part in the study. The time spent practicing physical activity among the participants was wide-ranging, with the shortest being 1 month and the longest 7 years.

4.2 Inclusion criteria:

S Belonging to the institution's gymnastics group;

S Is regularly registered with the Institute;

S Have a minimum attendance of 10 weeks

S Be able to practice physical activity by presenting a medical certificate.

4.3 Exclusion criteria:

S Elderly people with dementia;

S Seniors who practice gymnastics more than 4 times a week, including Tuesdays and Thursdays;

S Elderly people with severe osteoarticular and locomotion impairment,

These criteria will be accessed from the participant themselves through direct questioning by the researchers before the program begins.

4.4 Instruments used

Questionnaires:

S Personal identification;

S Basic Activities of Daily Living (KATZ, 1963);

S Instrumental Activities of Daily Living (LAWTON, 1969);

Advanced activities of daily living (MELO, 2009).

Body Perception:

Silhouette Figure Scale for Body Image Assessment (STUNKARD,

1983 adapted by KAKESHITA, 2008).

Muscular strength:

J Upper limbs - Elbow flexion (RIKLI; JONES, 1999);

J Lower limbs - 30" chair lift test (YAMAUCHI et al., 2005; ROGERS et al., 2003; RIKLI; JONES, 1999).

Flexibility:

S Sit and reach test (MATSUDO, 2010).

Aerobic endurance:

S 2-minute walk in place test (RIKLI; JONES, 1999).

Balance:

J Balance with visual control (MATSUDO, 2010).

1- The Katz index contains 6 questions relating to self-care activities. The person assessed must say whether they perform the activities questioned: without assistance, with minimal assistance or with total assistance. We score the alternative marked without assistance, and at the end we add up the points **(Appendix II).**

2- Scale of Instrumental Activities of Daily Living proposed by Lawton1(969), containing 7 questions with 3 alternatives: able to perform the activity alone, able to perform the activity with assistance or unable to perform the activity, in the end we scored only the alternative corresponding to á performing the activity alone and added it up **(Appendix II).**

3- Inventory of Advanced Activities of Daily Living, a questionnaire created by Melo (2009) adapted for this research, 12 questions referring to the frequency of performance of Advanced

Activities of Daily Living (AADLs) with three response options: Never done, stopped doing or still doing **(Annex III).**

Flowchart

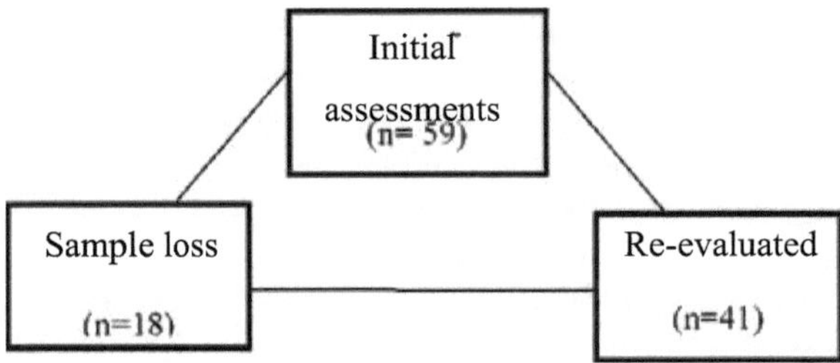

Figure 1- Project flowchart

We started the project with 59 elderly people, and during the 3 months of the intervention we lost 18, which represents a 30% sample loss. The cause of sample loss in this population is great, because at this stage of life medical consultations are more frequent and pathologies appear frequently, thus preventing regular physical activity.

4.4.1 Flexibility - Sit and reach tests

Material: the standard sit and reach test bench (Well bench).

To perform the test, the individual sits on the floor with their legs outstretched and their feet against the wooden bench, hip-width apart and arms outstretched. At the command "attention now", the test taker is instructed to flex their torso and move straight ahead, sliding their hands along the measuring tape which will be glued to the bench, until they reach the furthest point, without flexing their knee. Three attempts are made and the best value obtained is taken into account for the calculation.

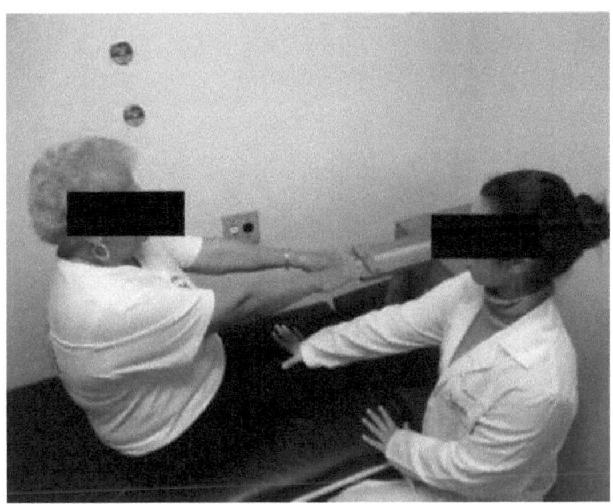

Figure 2- Flexibility test

4.4.2 Balance with visual control:

Materials: stopwatch and a place that offers a fixed point for viewing.

The person being tested stands with their hands on their waist and is told to look at a fixed point (a figure stuck to the wall) and bend the knee of one of their legs, forming a 90° angle, and try to hold this position for at least 30 seconds. The assessor remains at the subject's side, activating the stopwatch at the words of command and stopping at the first contact of the foot with the floor, or of the hands on a support placed in front of the subject. If the subject manages to hold the position for 30 seconds, the stopwatch is stopped at the end of this time and the subject is allowed to rest. Three attempts are made and the average in seconds is calculated.

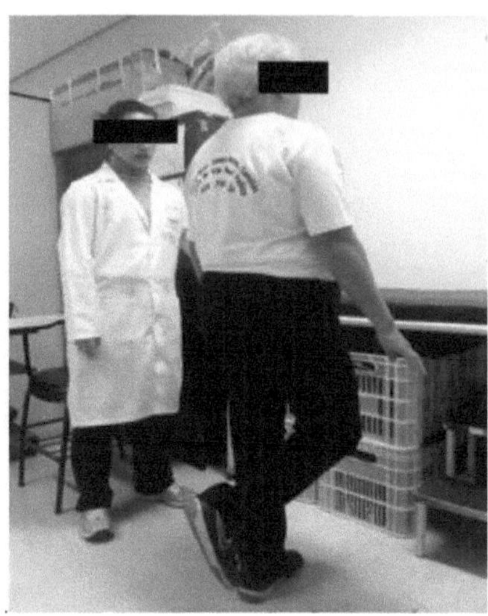

Figure 3- Balance test

4.4.3 Upper limb muscle strength - Elbow flexion

Materials: stopwatch, straight-backed or hinged chair (without arms), hand weights or dumbbells weighing 2 kg for women and 4 kg for men.

The test subject is seated on a chair, with their back straight against the backrest and their feet flat on the floor, with the dominant side of their body near the side edge of the chair. The weight is held at the side with the dominant hand closed. The test begins with the arm extended downwards at the side of the chair, perpendicular to the floor. At the *"attention now"* signal, the test taker turns their palm upwards while flexing their arm, fully completing the angle of movement, then returns to the starting position with the elbow fully extended. The assessor should be kneeling next to the subject, placing their fingers in the middle of the subject's bicep region to prevent the arm from moving and ensure that the full flexion movement is made. The subject will be encouraged to perform as many flexion movements as possible within 30 seconds.

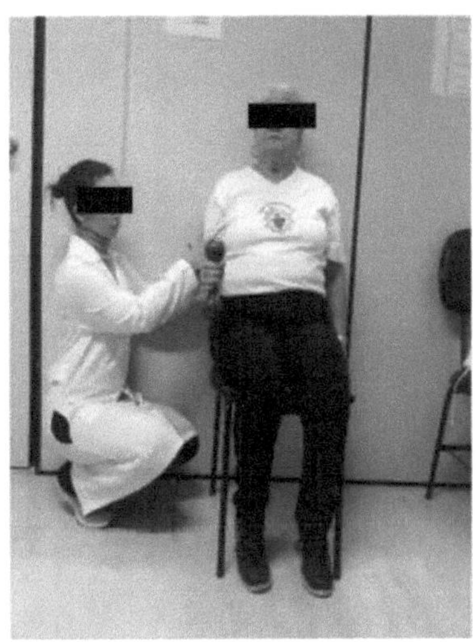

Figure 4- Elbow flexion

4.4.4 Lower limb muscle strength - Get up from chair in 30" *Materials*: stopwatch, straight-backed chair without arms, with an approximate height of 43 cm. For safety reasons, the chair remained against the wall to prevent it from moving during the test.

The test subject remained seated on the chair, with their back straight and their feet flat on the floor. His arms were crossed against his chest. At the *"attention, now"* signal, the subject stood up and then returned to a fully seated position. The subject was instructed to sit down completely as many times as possible in 30 seconds. If the participant was more than halfway through the movement at the end of the 30 seconds, it was counted as a complete movement.

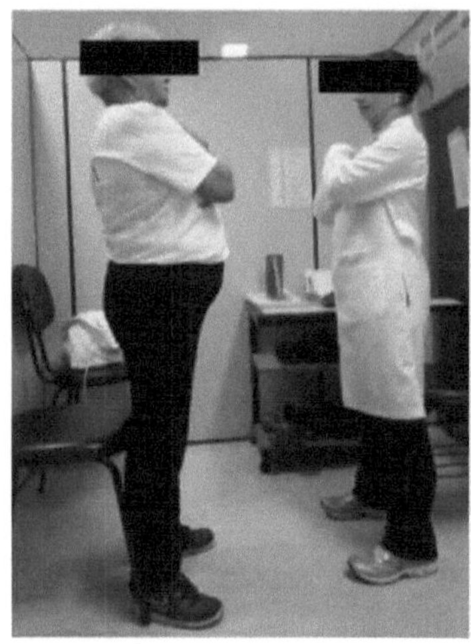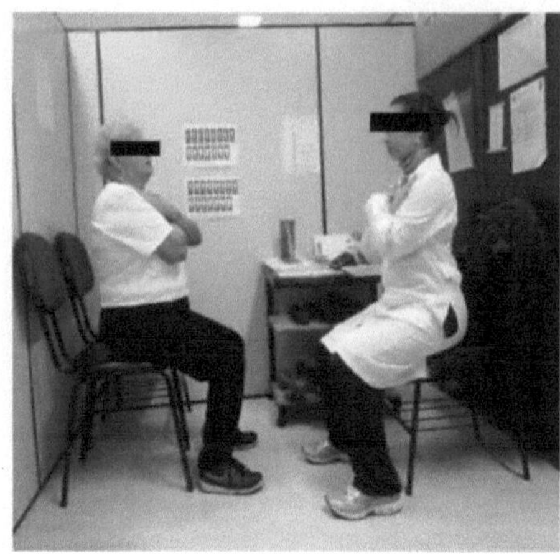

Figure 5 and 6 - 30-second chair stand and sit tests

4.4.5 Aerobic endurance - 2-minute walk test *Materials:* stopwatch, measuring tape and tape measure.

The minimum appropriate knee height to perform the step for each participant is at the level of the midpoint between the patella and the iliac crest. This point can be determined using a tape measure or simply by stretching a piece of string from the patella to the iliac crest, which is folded in half to determine the midpoint. To monitor the correct height of the knee when striding, you can use books placed on an adjacent table or a ruler attached to a chair or a piece of masking tape affixed to the wall. At the *"attention now"* signal, the participant starts bending their knees, simulating a stride (without running), without leaving their seat, starting with their right leg, completing as many strides as possible within the 2-minute time limit. Although the knees must be raised to the correct height to count the number of strides, the assessor only counts the number of times the right knee reaches the determined height. The assessor should stand to the side of the person being tested, stimulating their strides, and should warn them when 30 seconds have elapsed before the end of the test.

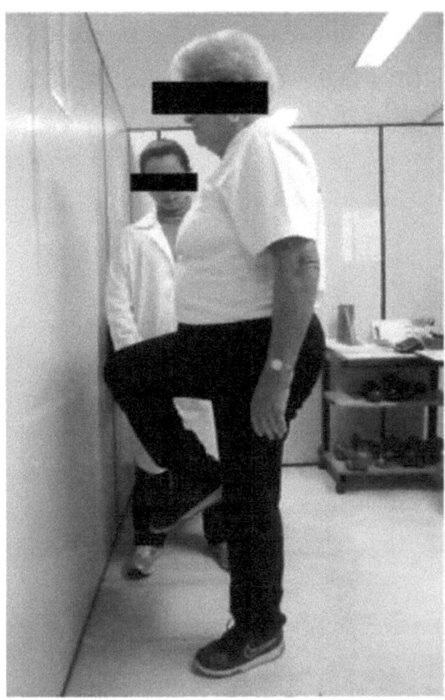

Figure 7- 2-minute walk in place test

4.4.6 Silhouette Scale for Brazilian Adults:

Material: silhouette scale for Brazilian adults.

Initially proposed by Stunkard (1983) and adapted and validated for the Brazilian population by Kakeshita (2009), the Adult Silhouette Scale consists of 15 figures of each gender, "presented on individual plastic cards, 6.5 cm wide by 12.5 cm high, with the figure centered on a black background and surrounded by a margin of 0.5 cm equidistant from the edges and the card" (KAKESHITA, 2009). These figures have no facial details or disproportionate shapes, with progressive variations in the scale of measurements, from the thinnest figure to the largest, with the average BMI (Body Mass Index) ranging from 12 to 47.5 kg/m2 (KAKESHITA, 2009). The application of the Kakeshita Silhouette Scale (2009) consists of arranging the 15 independent cards in ascending order, from silhouette 1 to 15, for the individuals to observe. The subject is then asked to point to the silhouette that is closest to their current body image (Real Silhouette). The assessor should then write down the number of the card indicated. They are then asked to define which silhouette is closest to the body they would like to have (Ideal Silhouette) (CAMPANA; TAVARES, 2009). Once these procedures have been carried out, the degree of body (in)satisfaction will be assessed by calculating the difference between the Ideal Silhouette (SI) and the Real Silhouette (SR). The greater this difference, the greater the degree of (in)satisfaction with the CI (CAMPANA; TAVARES, 2009).

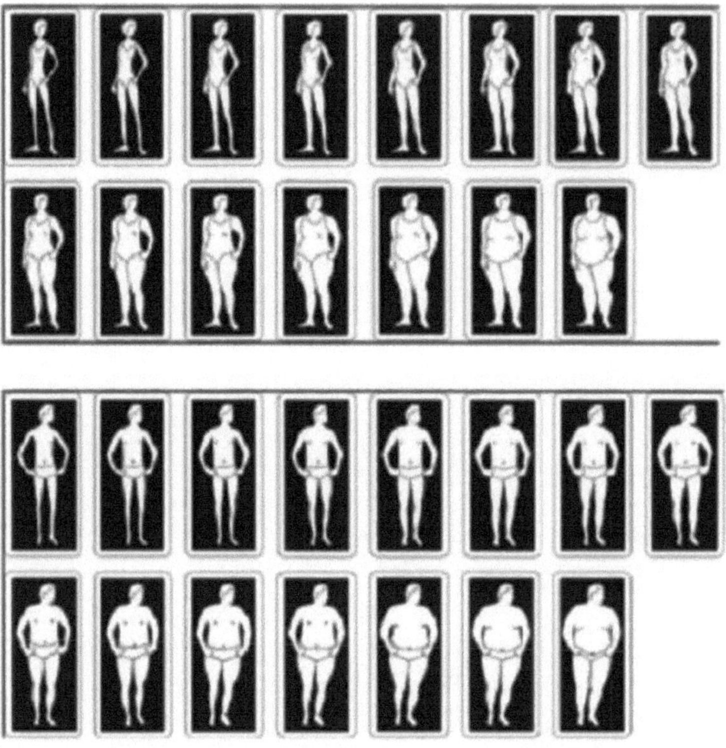

Figure 8- Silhouette Figure Scale for adults, female and male (KAKESHITA 2008).

5.   ETHICAL CONSIDERATIONS

This work will be submitted to the Research Ethics Committee through the Brazil Platform Registration, following the guidelines and norms that regulate research involving human beings, approved by Resolution no. 196, of October 10, 1996, of the National Health Council. Data collection will only begin after approval by the CEP.

All the participants in the study had access to the informed consent form (ICF), which was presented to them respecting all ethical conditions.

6.   STATISTICAL ANALYSIS

For the statistical analysis of the data, all the tests were analyzed using descriptive statistics (mean ± standard deviation). The inferential analyses of the neuromotor tests were carried out using ANOVA (Analysis of Variance with Repeated Measures). The significance level adopted was 5% ($p \leq 0.05$).

7. RESULTS AND DISCUSSION

7.1 SUBJECTS

A questionnaire was used to characterize the sample. A total of 59 elderly people of both sexes were assessed, 53 women and 6 men with an average age of 68±4 years.

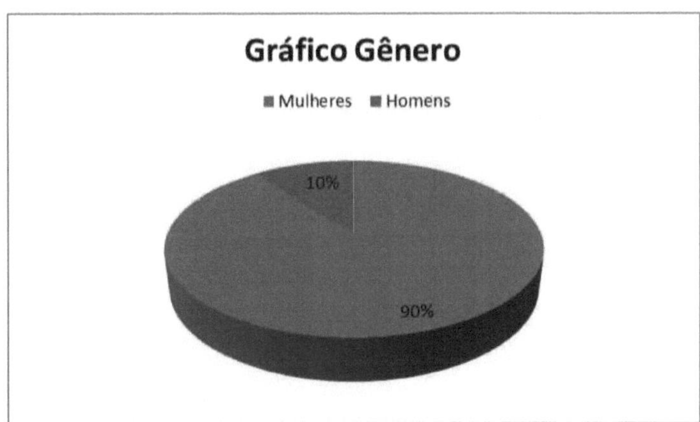

Figure 9. Graphical representation of the genus.

We observed in the sample that the level of education of the population studied was low, with 64% of individuals having studied up to elementary school, 29% having studied up to secondary school, 5% having studied up to higher education and 2% being illiterate **(Figures 10 and 11)**.

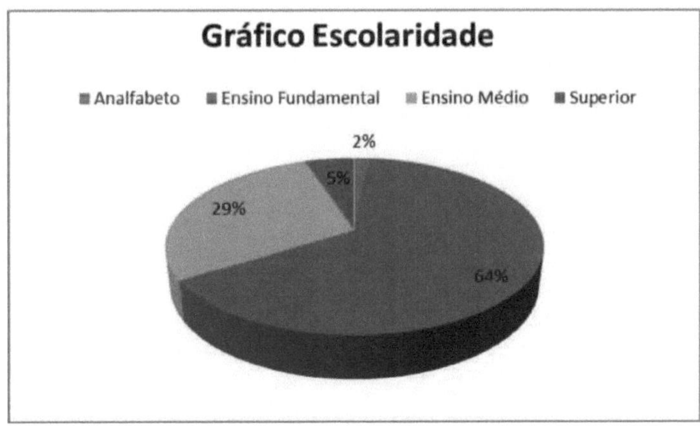

Figure 10. Graphical representation of education level.

With regard to marital status, the number of widowed individuals predominated, as did the number of married people.

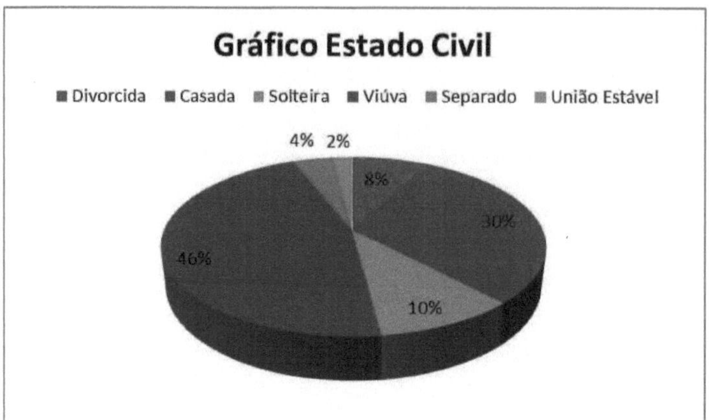

Figure 11. Graphical representation of marital status.

With regard to the profession held by the elderly, 56 were retired and only 3 were still working. The individuals had a variety of occupations, the most common being housewife, followed by industrial worker and seamstress.

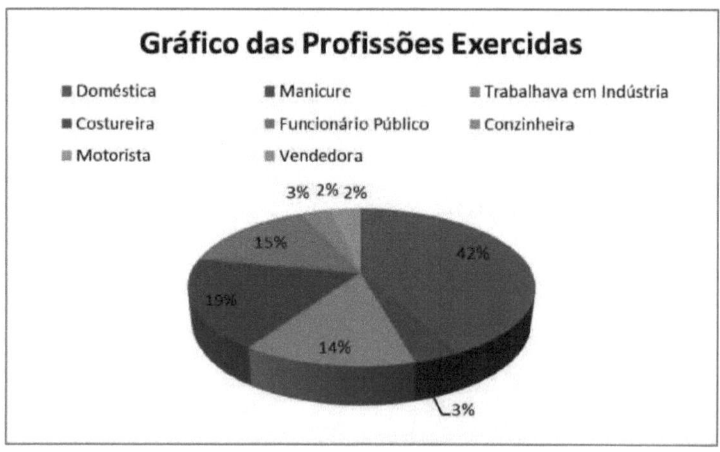

Figure 12. Graphical representation of professions held.

7.2 DAILY LIFE scales

Using the questionnaires related to activities of daily living, we can see that on the Kartz scale, representing basic activities of daily living, 33 elderly people were independent (56%),

26 were partially dependent (44%) and none were totally dependent on basic activities of daily living. On the Lawton scale representing instrumental activities of daily living, we found 5 independent (8%), 43 partially dependent (73%) and 11 totally dependent (19%). On the Base scale, which represents advanced activities of daily living, we found 47 independent (80%), 11 partially dependent (18%) and 1 totally dependent (2%). As can be seen in table 1.

Table 1 - Values for the number of elderly people with a degree of dependence in activities of daily living and their percentages.

	Kartz scale	□ %	Lawton Scale	□ %	Base	□ %
Independent	33	56%	5	8%	47	80%
Partially Dependent	26	44%	43	73%	11	18%
Dependent Total	0	0%	11	19%	1	2%

7.3 FLEXIBILITY

When analyzing Flexibility, the two groups did not show statistical differences, as they showed similarities in the maximum cm reached after the 3 attempts to flex the trunk at the most distal point possible in the sitting position, as we can see in table 2.

Table 2 - Mean values, standard deviation and □ % of the Aexibility test.

Flexibility	Before	After	□ %
	23±9	23±9	0%

P= 0.8986

In his study, Rebelatto et al (2005) reported that with ageing there is a decrease in the neuromuscular system, such as the loss of flexibility which is associated with the elasticity of the tendons, ligaments and capsule which in turn decrease with age due to collagen deficiency, determining that during active life, adults lose something like 8-10 cm of flexibility in the lumbar region and the hip, when measured using the sit and reach test, the same applied in this study, only with a different nomenclature. Therefore, despite the fact that the flexibility test showed no statistically significant differences, we can say that flexibility was maintained in the elderly studied, even though it tended to decrease.

These authors subjected 32 elderly women aged 60-80 to a physical activity program focused on manual strength and flexibility, lasting 2 years (58 weeks more specifically) and found no significant differences, only the maintenance of flexibility, thus agreeing with our evidence. In the literature review by Rogério et al (2008) on training and flexibility, it was observed that flexibility has a reversibility effect. A study carried out with adolescents showed that within 24 hours the flexibility gain obtained by training disappeared, i.e. it returned to the same level as before. The authors therefore argue that flexibility training should be done on a daily basis and point out that for the elderly, the ideal is to combine flexibility and strength training. In dance classes we hardly ever combine strength and flexibility training, and our classes were only held twice a week.

The dance program performed by the elderly in this study didn't include much stretching, we didn't do specific exercises for the lumbar spine, such as exercises on mats with the trunk thrust forward, all the stretching was done standing up or on a chair and the time spent in class was short, which may justify the findings.

7.4 BALANCE WITH VISUAL CONTROL

In relation to the balance test with visual control, whose objective was to measure the ability to remain static with only one support (right or left foot) for as long as possible, the longest time being 30", we can observe an improvement in time of 15% in relation to before and after the dance program, thus showing significant changes, as described in table 3.

Table 3 - Mean values, standard deviation and □ % of balance with visual control.

Balance	Before	After	□ %
	22±9	25±7	15%

P= 0,0032

In agreement with our findings, Aveiro et al (2004), in their study of osteoporotic women aged 60-74, found an improvement in static balance after physical training for 12 consecutive weeks at a frequency of three times a week and lasting one hour.

Jarek et al (2010) associate the positive gain in balance with positive changes in the muscular strength of the lower limbs, because when we perform resistance exercises to obtain muscular strength, we recruit a greater number of type II fibers (which are the fibers responsible for rapid contraction), that is, they are responsible for reaction time and concrete responses in emergency situations, thus directly interfering with balance. The same authors found a statistically significant improvement using the Berg scale in the static and dynamic balance of 10 elderly people who underwent a bodybuilding program with a minimum practice time of 4 months and a frequency of 3 times a week.

Another study that assessed static and dynamic balance using the Berg scale and found significant data was by Gomes; Wischneski and Rox (2012). They assessed 46 elderly people of both sexes and divided them into 4 groups: a control group, a group that performed resistance exercises, a group that performed stretching exercises and a group that mixed resistance exercises and stretching. The program lasted 12 weeks, twice a week. All the groups that underwent the physical activity programs improved, with a higher level of performance in the group that mixed stretching exercises with resistance exercises. Pereira (2012) found positive changes in dynamic balance using the *Tandem Walk Test*. His study evaluated the effect of a program of rhythmic activities for 12 weeks, twice a week, very similar to this study and his data corroborate those observed in this study.

In this way, our results reinforce previous studies showing that a dance program with activities similar to those of daily life promotes significant improvements in static balance in individuals over 60 years of age.

7.5 MUSCLE STRENGTH

Lower limbs

In the assessment of lower limb muscle strength using the 30-second chair stand test, the aim of which was to perform the greatest number of movements (stand and sit) in a 30-second interval, we found a significant increase of 25% in the number of repetitions, so the protocol had a positive effect on motor performance in this test, as shown in Table 4.

Table 4 - Mean values, standard deviation and □% of the lower limb muscle strength test.

Lower limb strength	Before	After	□ %
	10±2	13±2	25%

P= <0.0001

Upper limbs

When we analyzed the muscle strength of the upper limbs using the elbow flexion test, the aim of which was to perform as many arm flexion and extension movements as possible in

30 seconds, we noticed a significant difference in the number of movements performed, so the dance program had a positive effect on muscle strength, as shown in Table 5.

Table 5 - Mean values, standard deviation and □ % of the upper limb muscle strength test.

Upper limb strength	Before	After	□ %
	12±2	15±2	24%

P= <0.0001

The significant results in the lower and upper limb muscle strength tests in the present study are in agreement with those obtained in the study by Alves et al (2005) who evaluated 74 elderly women over 60 years of age, who took part in aquatic exercise classes for 12 weeks, twice a week for 45 minutes, with a 6% increase in lower limb muscle strength after the intervention, and 9% in the upper limbs, the authors used the Rikli and Jones test battery which measures the level of physical fitness of the elderly through some variables.

Mazo et al (2012) in their cross-sectional study with 891 elderly people, which aimed to assess physical fitness (coordination, agility, dynamic balance, muscular strength endurance) used the American Alliance for Health, Physical Education, Recreation and Dance (AHPERD) test battery for the elderly, observed positive and significant results in all variables in the group that practiced physical activity even with osteoarticular diseases, collaborating with the significant data of Aveiro et al (2004) who found an improvement in quadriceps muscle strength of 25% in osteoporotic women after a physical training program.

According to Lynch et al (1999) the muscle mass of the lower limbs seems to be more affected by the ageing process than that of the upper limbs, mainly due to the reduction in the level of physical activity which affects the extension of the lower limbs more, and due to the compensation of strength in the upper limb due to weakness in the legs, because the elderly mostly use their upper limbs when they stand up for example, this determines greater use of the upper limbs consequently maintaining muscle strength. However, Amaral et al (2012), after evaluating 22 women with an average age of 68±6 years by means of maximum isometric effort, did not find statistically significant differences in the strength of the lower and upper limbs; however, the data found suggest a steeper decline in the lower limbs. Our study found a 25% gain in lower limb strength and a 24% gain in upper limb strength, which is not in line with the studies mentioned above.

Another piece of evidence was in the study by Jarek et al (2010) who also found statistically significant differences in lower and upper limb muscle strength in the elderly who took part in a bodybuilding program. Pereira (2012), on the other hand, did not find any significant results when evaluating upper limb muscle strength in the elderly who took part in a rhythmic activity program using the hand press test.

It is worth noting that most of the studies cited measured the maximum load for each individual to perform the 1RM resistance exercises. In this study, to gain strength in the lower limbs, there was no overload; the exercises were performed with the body's own weight, while for the upper limbs we used a chair in the last month to simulate the barbell curl exercise to strengthen the biceps, but all the participants used the same material.

7.6 AEROBIC ENDURANCE

2-minute walk in place test

With regard to the aerobic endurance test, the aim of which was to measure the number of steps taken simulating walking and raising the knee to the hip for 2 minutes, we observed a notable and significant improvement in the number of steps taken for 2 minutes before and after the protocol, as shown in Table 6.

Table 6 - Mean values, standard deviation and □ % of the aerobic endurance test.

Resistance Aerobics	Before	After	□ %
	70±16	85±2	21%

P= <0.0001

Perceived exertion in the aerobic endurance test

To analyze the perception of effort, we used a table with increasing numbers, which represented the effort exerted in the endurance test. The evaluator asked the participant how they measured the effort exerted in the test: a lot of effort, effort, moderate effort, I didn't exert myself (we changed the question to tiredness if necessary). There was no significant difference, so we can say that the participant was able to perform the aerobic endurance test more efficiently, increasing the number of steps without, however, trying harder or feeling more tired, and this observation favored the result obtained in the endurance test, as we can see in table 7.

Table 7 - Mean values, standard deviation and □ % of the perceived exertion test in the aerobic endurance test.

Perception of Effort	Before	After	□ %
	13±1	13±1	0%

P= 0.5938

To assess aerobic endurance, balance, flexibility and lower and upper limb strength, Penha et a.l (2012) used the same test as this study and generally observed significant changes in all the variables, including aerobic endurance, reinforcing our findings. The authors found significant differences of 16.4% to 30.0% in aerobic endurance after an aerobic exercise program lasting 50 minutes twice a week for 3.4 years and months.

Mazo et. al. (2012) in their study using the AHPERD test battery for the elderly, observed positive and significant results in the aerobic endurance variable by calculating the percentile score. Cipriani et al. (2010) used the same *American Alliance for Health, Physical Education, Recreation and Dance* test battery and analyzed 225 elderly women who took part in a physical exercise program (folk dance), observing a significant improvement in the agility/dynamic balance variables. Pereira's (2012) data also showed significant results using the test of sitting and getting up from a chair and moving around the house.

In the literature, we didn't find any more expressive results for aerobic endurance in specific; the studies evaluated it when it was combined with other tests, as we can see. However, our results show a significant change in aerobic endurance after the dance program with movements similar to activities of daily living, thus highlighting the benefit of dance in the cardiorespiratory conditioning of elderly individuals. We believe that these results are related to the fast movements and changes of direction that dance requires.

7.7 BODY IMAGE

Table 8 and 9 show that there were no statistically significant differences between the actual and ideal silhouette before and after the dance program. However, there was a decrease in the number of body image figures chosen before and after. This means that before the dance program the figure chosen by the elderly to represent them had a larger silhouette compared to the figures chosen after the dance program.

Real

Table 8 - Mean values, standard deviation and □ % of the real body image test.

Real body image	Before	After	%
	10±2	9±2	-5%

P= 0.1268

Ideal

Table 9 - Mean values, standard deviation and □ % of the ideal body image test.

Ideal body image	Before	After	□ %
	8±2	7±2	-6%

P= 0.1687

In the study by Damasceno et al (2006) which reviewed the literature on body image from childhood to old age, they concluded that in the ageing phase, in addition to the question of physical appearance, the decline in functionality affects satisfaction with the body. Moreira and Silva (2013) share this view and found that body image and bodily changes represent defining factors in the perception of the ageing process. When they questioned 40 elderly people aged between 60 and 77, they found that more than half of those interviewed considered body image to be the factor that best announces ageing. In this way we can see how the issue of body image is still strongly rooted in the elderly population.

Machado, Sudo and Pinto (2010) assessed the body image of 53 elderly women living in a long-stay institution using the Sturkard silhouette scale and found that 49.1% of the women were satisfied with their bodies, 35.8% were dissatisfied and wanted to reduce their weight and 15.1% wanted to increase their weight. Other studies that assessed body image using the same instrument were Matsudo et al (2007) and Pereira (2012), who found that elderly women who practiced physical activities were more satisfied with their body image. Pereira (2008) found that of the 62 elderly women who had been practicing water aerobics for at least 5 years, 72% were dissatisfied with their body image due to being overweight.

In our results, we found no positive changes regarding body image in the elderly. We suggest that these findings are related to the incessant search for the beautiful body that society imposes all the time, especially through the media, affecting people more and more, so that they feel incapable of achieving the ideal body on display. It would be no different with the elderly population, who are vulnerable to feeling devalued because of the disabilities caused by the ageing process. Thus, the elderly in this study, even though they were part of the dance program, did not have higher levels of satisfaction with their body image.

8.   LIMITATIONS OF THE STUDY

The small number of participants in the survey, the lack of a more comprehensive daily life questionnaire for the active population and the low number of men in the study.

9. CONCLUSION

However, we can conclude that the dance program with movements that simulate the activities of daily life of the elderly promoted the maintenance and expressive and significant gains in the motor functions of the elderly. This showed improvements in their activities of daily living. It is worth pointing out that physical activity is an effective element in maintaining health, bringing us various benefits, both physical, as detected in this study, and psychological, which are subjective improvements: a sense of well-being, pleasure, self-esteem. For the elderly, it is therefore a fundamental tool for remaining independent for as long as possible.

10.   BIBLIOGRAPHICAL REFERENCES

AMARAL,J.F; CASTRO, E.A; MANCINI,M; DOIMO,L.A; NOVOJÛNIORJ.L. **Rate of development of upper and lower limb muscle strength in elderly women.** Motricidade, v.8,n.2,p.445-461, 2012.

ALVES, J.E.D. **A transiçâçâo demogràfica e a janela de oportunidade.** Sao Paulo: Fernand Braudel Institute of World Economics; 2008.

ALVES,V.R; MOTA,J; COSTA,C.D.M; ALVES, B.G.J. **Aptidao fisica relacionada á saù de idosos: influência da hidroginâstica.** Rev. bras. Med. Espote, v.10,n. 1, Jan/Feb, 2004.

ASKEVOLD, F. Measuring Body Image. **Psychoter. Psychosom**. v. 26, p. 71-77, 1975.

AVEIRO, M.C; NAVEGA, M.T; GRANITO, R.N; RENNÓ, A.C.M; OISHI, J.

Effects of a physical activity program on balance and quadriceps muscle strength in osteoporotic women aiming to improve quality of life. Rev. bras.Ci.e Mov.; 12(3): 33-38.) 2004.

BORGES, D.R.M; MOREIRA, K.A**. Influências da pràtica de actividades fisicas na terceira idade: estudo comparativo dos níveis de autonomia para o desempenho nas AVDs e AIVDs entre idosos ativos fisicamente e idosos sedentàrios.** Revista: Motriz, Rio Claro, v.15 n.13 p. 562-573, jul./set, 2009.

CAMPANA, A.N.N.B; TAVARES, M.C.G.C.F. Avaliação da Imagem CorporaLInstrumentos e diretrizes para pesquisa. Revista Forte - Sao Paulo 2009.

CARLA ET AL. **Aging and dance: analysis of scientific production in the Virtual Health Library.** *Rev. bras. geriatr. gerontol.* [online]. 2013, vol.16, n.1, pp. 191-199. ISSN 1809-9823.

CIPRIANI, N. C. S. et al. **Functional** fitness of **elderly women practicing physical activities.** Rev Bras Cineantropom Desempenho Hum. v. 12, n. 12, p. 106-111, 2010.

FITNESS COOPERATIVE. Needs and Restrictions of the Elderly. How does the body age? January, 2009. Accessed at http://www.cdof.com.br/idosos1.htm. Last accessed on 09/09/2013.

CORRÊA D.A.; OLIVEIRA, S.C.; BASSANI, A.M. **Being beyond the walls: phenomenology of freedom for institutionalized elderly.** Rev. abordagem gestalt. vol.24 no.2 Goiânia maio/go. 2018.

COUTO, D. V. T; OVANDO, K. M. L. **Psychomotor activities as an intervention in the functional performance of hospitalized elderly people. Revista:** Mundo saùde (Impr.) (1995); 34(2): 176-182 Apr.-Jun. 2010. graf, tab.

DAMASCENO, V.O; VIANNA, V.R.A; VIANNA, J.M; LACIO, M.; LIMA, J.R.P.; NOVAES, J.S. **Body image and ideal body.** R. bras. Ci e Mov.; 14(1): 87-96, 2006.

DUCA, D. F. G; HALLAL, C. P; SILVA, D. C. M. **Functional incapacity for basic and instrumental activities of daily living in the elderly.** Revista Saùde Pùblica, Pelotas, Rio Grande do Sul, 2009.

FONSECA, C.C. **Body Schema, Body Image and motivational aspects in ballroom dancing.** Master's dissertation, Physical Education - Sao Judas Tadeu University, Sao Paulo, 2008.

FREITAS, M. C., QUEIROZ, T. A., & SOUSA, J. A. V. **O significado da velhice e da experiência de envelhecer para os idosos.** Revista da Escola de Enfermagem da USP, 44(2), 407-412. Guimaraes, I.; Carneiro, M. H, 2010.

United Nations Population Fund. Executive Summary. **Ageing in the 21st Century: Celebration and Challenge.** New York; 2012.

GOLIN, A.F. Dança e **Movimento: um significado para pessoa portadora de deficiência visual.** Revista Virtual Beijamin Constant, Rio de Janeiro, v.8, n.21, p. 3-5, 2005.

GOMES,S.R.A; WISCHNESKI,P; ROX, R. **Whether or not to associate stretching with resistance exercise to improve balance in the elderly?** Biblioteca virtual de saù Lillacs Acta fisiâtrica, bases.bireme.br 2011.

IBGE, 2008. **Projection of the Population of Brazil by Sex and Age: 1980-2050 - Revised 2008** (On-line).Available athttp://www.ibge.gov.br/home/estatistica/populacao/projecao_da_populacao/2008/def

ault.shtm. Accessed on: 20/08/2013

JAREK,C; OLIVEIRA, H.M;NANTES, R.W; ULBRICHT, L; MASCARENHAS, G.P.L. **Anthropometric comparison, muscle strength and balance between elderly bodybuilders and non-bodybuilders.** Passa Fundo,v.7,n.2,p.173-180, May/Aug.2010.

KAKESHITA, I.S. **Adaptation and validation of Silhouette Scales for Brazilian children and adults.** PhD Thesis - Faculty of Philosophy. University of Sao Paulo, Ribeirao Preto, 2008.

KAKESHITA, I. S. et al. **Construction and Test-Retest Reliability of Brazilian Silhouette Scales for Adults and Children.** Psicologia: Teoria e Pràtica, v. 25, n. 2, p. 263-270, April-June 2009.

KALACHE, A. **The world is ageing: it is imperative to create a social solidarity pact.** Ciênc Saùde Coletiva;13(4):1107-11, 2008.

KATZ S, FORD AB, MOSKOWITZ RW, **Jackson BA, Jaffe MW. Studies of Illness in the Aged. the Index of Adl**: a Standardized Measure of Biological.

LAWTON MP, BRODY EM. **Assessment of older people: self-maintaining and instrumental activities of daily living.** *Gerontologist.* 1969;9(3):179-86.

LIMA- COSTA MF, MATOS DL, CAMARGOS VP, MACINKO J. **Ten-year trends in the health conditions of elderly Brazilians: evidence from the National Household Sample Survey (1998, 2003, 2008).** Ciênc Saùde Coletiva;16:3689-96, 2011

LYNCH,N.A; METTER,E.J; LINDLE,R.S; FOZARD,J.L; TOBIN,J.D; ROY,T.A, HURLEY,B.F. **Muscle quality-I: Age-associated differences between arm leg muscle groups.** Journal of applied physiology, 86(1), 188-194 1999.

MACHADO,C.D; SUDO,N; PINTO,G.H.A. **Imagem corporal de idosas que residem em uma instituição de longa permanência de Porto Alegre -RS.** Ceres: nutriçao e saùde; 5(3),139-148, 2010.

MARCIANO, V; BARBOSA, R.A. **Protótipo do Belo: Imagem Real x Imagem Corporal.** Revista Pulsar - v. 1, n. 2, 2009.

MATSUDO,F.R; VELARDI,M; BRANDAO,F.R.M; MIRANDA,J.D.L.M. **Imagem Corporal de idosas e atividade fisica.** Rev. Mackenzie de educaçao fisica e esporte, 6(1) 37-43, 2007.

MATSUDO, S. M. **Assessment of the elderly: Physical and Functional.** 3ª ed. Santo Amaro: Gràfica Mali, Sao Paulo, 2010.

MAZO,Z.G; SACOMORRI, C; KRUG, R.D.R; BENEDETII,B.R.T. **Physical fitness, physical exercise and osteoarticular diseases in the elderly.** Rev. Bràs. Ativ. e Saùde, Pelotas R/S agos. 2012.

MELO, D. M. **Frailty, performance of advanced activities of daily living and perceived health in elderly people treated at a geriatric outpatient clinic.** Master's dissertation in Gerontology, Faculty of Medical Sciences, State University of Campinas - UNICAMP, Sao Paulo, 2009.

MINAYO, M. C. S.; COIMBRA, J. C. E. A. Introduction. **Between Freedom and Dependence: reflections on the social phenomenon of ageing.** In. M. C. S. Minayo; C. E. A. Coimbra Junior (Orgs.), Anthropology, Health and Ageing (pp. 11-24). Rio de Janeiro: Fiocruz, 2002.

Miranda, D.; Morais, G.; Mendes, G.; Cruz, A.; Silva, A.; Lucia, A. **Brazil's ageing population: current and future social challenges and consequences.** Revista Brasileira de Geriatria e Gerontologia, vol. 19, no. 3, julio-septiembre, pp. 507-519, Rio de Janeiro, 2016.

MOREIRA,O.D.J; SILVA,D.M.J. **Body image and aging from the perspective of professors at a Brazilian university.** Salud e Sociedad, v.4,n.2, p.136-144, agos/2013.

PENHA, L.C.J; PIÇARRO,C.D.I; NETO,B.D.L.T. **Evoluçao da aptida física e capacidade funcional de mulheres ativas acima de 50 anos de idade de acordo com a idade cronològica, na cidade de Santos.** Rev. Ciência e Saùde Coletiva, 17(1):245- 253,2012.

PEREIRA, E. S. **Effects of a program of rhythmic exercises that simulate activities of daily living in the elderly.** Master's dissertation, Physical Education - Sao Judas Tadeu University, Sao Paulo, 2012.

PEREIRA,F.E; TEXEIRA,S.C; BORGATTO,F.A; DARONCO,E.S.L. **Relationship between different anthropometric indicators and body image perception in active elderly women**. Rev. Psiq Clin, 36(2):54:9, 2009.

REBELATTO, J.R; CALVO, J. I; OREJUELA, J.R.; PORTILLO, J.C.. **Influence of a long-term physical activity program on manual muscle strength and body flexibility in elderly women.** Revista brasileira fisioterapia, vol.10, n., p. 127-132, 2006.

RIBEIRO, R.G; DOMINGUES, O.D; SILVA, A.V. **Flexibility training and its relationship with activities of daily living in aging: a review study.** Revista brasileira de ciências da saùde, ano III, n.17, jul/set 2008.

RIKLI, R.; JONES, J. **Functional fitness normative scores for community-residing older adults**, ages 60-94. J Aging Phys Act. v. 7, p. 162-181, 1999.

SEGHETO, J.K. **Effect of proprioceptive stimuli on the Body Perception of adult individuals.** Master's Degree in Physical Education - Sao Judas Tadeu University, Sao Paulo, 2010.

SILVA, A. J. D., SCORSOLINI, C.F., & SANTOS, M. A. **Elderly in long-term care facilities: development, living conditions and health.** Psicologia: Reflexao Critica, 26 (4), 820-830, 2013.

STUNKARD, A. J.; SORENSEN, T.; SHULSINGUER, F. Use of the Danish adoption register for the study of obesity and thinness. **Research Publication - Association for Research in Nervous and Mental Disorders,** v. 60, 1983.

TAVARES, M.C.G.C.F. **A imagem corporal e a dança**. Revista Conexoes, Campinas, n.6, p. 10-22, 2001.

TAVARES, M.C.C. **Body Image: Concept and Development**. Sao Paulo: Manole.2003.

THOMAS, J.R; NELSON, J.K; SILVERMAM, S.J. **Research methods in physical activity**. 5.ed. Porto Alegre: Artmed, 2007.

THURM, E.B. **Effects of Chronic Pain in High-Performance Athletes on Body Schema, Psychomotor Agility and Mood States.** Master's Degree in Physical Education - Sao Judas

Tadeu University, Sao Paulo, 2007.

YAMAUCHI, T. et al, **Effect of home-based well-rounded exercise in communitydwelling older adults.** J Sports Sci Med. v. 4, p. 563-571, 2005.

ANNEX I

Informed Consent Form

EU

.bearer of ID: ....I hereby declare that I have agreed to take part in the research project **Effects of a Dance Program with Characteristic Movements on Activities of Daily Living in the Elderly**, which will be carried out at the IPGG (Instituto Paulista de Geriatria e Gerontologia) located in the Sao Paulo region.

I am aware that my participation is not compulsory and that I can withdraw my consent at any time without any prejudice. I affirm that I have agreed to take part of my own free will, without receiving any financial incentive for the sole purpose of collaborating in the success of the research. I have been informed of the strictly academic aims of the study, which, in general terms, are to analyze the effects of a dance program with everyday movements on the functional response and body perception of the elderly. I was made aware of the risks and benefits of the research, which are possible embarrassment that may arise after the tests have been applied, and the benefit of having a better performance in activities of daily living, as well as obtaining information on how to improve my body perception.

I was also informed that the use of the information I provided is subject to the ethical standards for research involving human beings of the National Research Ethics Commission (CONEP) and that my individual information will be kept confidential.

This ICF is issued in two copies signed by the participant and the researcher, one copy for each.

Sao Paulo, _____2014.

Research subject

Daniela de Almeida Pontes

End. Praça Padre Aleixo Monteiro Mafra, 34Michele Maia Pontes

Cep: 080011-010

End. Praça Padre Aleixo Monteiro Mafra, 34

Tel: 2030-4035

Cep: : 080011-010Tel

: 2030-403

Identification/ Scales/ Tests

Name:Date of Birth

Age: _________________ Marital status: _________________

Education:Profession:

BASIC ACTIVITIES OF DAILY LIFE SCALE (Katz, 1963)

1. Bath

( ) does not receive assistance

( ) assistance for one part of the body

( ) doesn't bathe alone

2. Clothing

( ) dresses without assistance

( ) assistance with tying shoes

( ) assistance with dressing

3. Personal hygiene

( ) goes to the toilet without assistance

( ) receives assistance to go to the toilet

( ) doesn't go to the toilet for physiological eliminations

4. Transfer

( ) lies down, stands up and sits down without assistance

( ) lies down, stands up and sits down with assistance

( ) doesn't get out of bed

5. Continence

( ) Complete sphincter control (elimination of urine and feces)

( ) Occasional accidents

( ) supervision, catheter use or incontinent

6. Food

( ) without assistance

( ) assistance with cutting meat/butter into bread

( ) with assistance, or probes, or fluids

INSTRUMENTAL ACTIVITIES OF DAILY LIVING SCALE (LAWTON, 1969)

a) Telephone

( ) receives and makes calls without assistance

( ) call assistance or special telephone

( ) unable to use the phone

b) Travel

( ) travels alone

( ) travels exclusively accompanied

( ) unable to travel

c) Purchasing

( ) shopping, if transportation is provided

( ) goes shopping together

( ) incapable

e) Domestic work

( ) incapable

f) Medications

g) Money

( ) writes checks and pays bills

( ) assistance with checks and bills

( ) incapable

( ) unable to take it alone

d) Meal preparation

( ) plans and cooks complete meals

( ) only prepares small meals

( ) incapable

( ) heavy tasks

( ) light tasks, with help with heavy ones

( ) takes medication without assistance

( ) needs reminders or assistance

( ) unable to take it alone

ANNEX III

ADVANCED ACTIVITIES OF DAILY LIFE (Berlin Age Study, BASE)

I would like to know what your relationship is with the following activities?

	Never did	Stopped to do	Still does
Visiting other people's homes	(1)	(2)	(3)
Receiving visitors in your home	(1)	(2)	(3)
Going to church or temple for religious rituals or religiously-related social activities	(1)	(2)	(3)
Participate in a community center, University of the Third Age or a course	(1)	(2)	(3)
Attend social gatherings, parties or dances	(1)	(2)	(3)
Attend cultural events such as concerts, shows, exhibitions, plays or films at the cinema	(1)	(2)	(3)
Driving a car	(1)	(2)	(3)
Day trips out of town	(1)	(2)	(3)
Longer trips out of town or out of the country	(1)	(2)	(3)
Do voluntary work	(1)	(2)	(3)
Do paid work	(1)	(2)	(3)
Serving on the boards or councils of associations, clubs, schools, unions, cooperatives or community centers, or engaging in political activities	(1)	(2)	(3)

NEUROMOTOR ASSESSMENT

Trunk Flexibility (cm)

Attempt 1	Attempt 2	Attempt 3

Static equilibrium (seconds)

Time 1	Time 2	Time 3

Rise from Chair 30 seconds (repetitions)

Attempt

Elbow flexion 30 seconds (repetitions)

Attempt

Metabolic Assessment

Step 2 minutes - Reference: _______ cm

	30sec	60sec	90sec	120sec
Repetitions				
PSE				

BODY IMAGE TEST & BODY PERCEPTION

BMI:

IMCP	IMCI

PC:

Reference No.	Observations

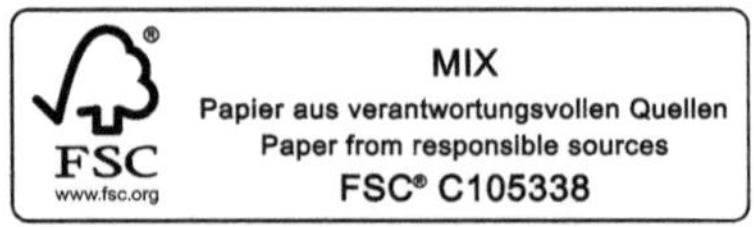